# Hip Replacement Surgery Advice From A Patient

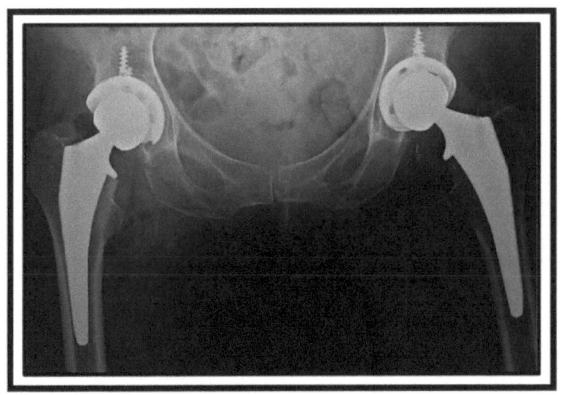

By Norma Rose
Copyright © 2023

Updated 03/30/2023

# TABLE OF CONTENTS

INTRODUCTION ..................................................................... 3

TRUST YOUR DOCTOR ........................................................... 5

BEFORE SURGERY .................................................................. 8
    Get Healthy ..................................................................... 8
    Schedule Dental & Doctor Visits ..................................... 8
    Get Your House Setup .................................................... 9
    Get the Tools You Will Need ........................................... 9
    Get Medications ............................................................ 10

A TOUR OF MY HOUSE ........................................................ 11
    Captain's Chair ............................................................. 12
    Office Desk ................................................................... 13
    Porta Potty ................................................................... 15
    Large Recliner .............................................................. 20
    Shower ......................................................................... 23
    Sink Setup .................................................................... 25
    Big Tools ...................................................................... 27
    Little Tools ................................................................... 29
    Tools For Dogs ............................................................. 35

TRAVELING TIPS ................................................................. 38

# Introduction

This book contains advice for people who plan to have hip replacement surgery. The advice is from me – an elderly female, who had two, separate hip replacement surgeries. Those with a similar profile will be more likely to find my advice helpful than those with a different profile. But, hopefully, everyone who is planning to have hip replacement surgery can benefit from my experience and advice.

I was 70-years-old when I had both hips replaced in two separate operations, three months apart. I had been hobbling around for several years (too long) before finally getting my hips replaced.

In addition to arthritic hips, I had some other health issues that made the surgery and recovery more difficult. I won't go into detail here, but the list includes: Previous right-knee reconstruction, total right-knee replacement, left-foot bunion, right-foot nerve damage, and scoliosis of the spine.

# Trust your doctor

Total hip replacement surgery is a fairly common and successful surgery. Do some online research, ask friends, and learn as much as you can about the procedure and the doctors available to you.

You will find many qualified doctors, in many locations, with different surgical approaches (e.g. anterior or posterior) and with different recovery philosophies (slow or fast). Depending on your situation, one approach might be more appropriate. I don't know, I'm not a doctor!

I think the best thing to do is to find a good doctor and trust him or her to use the right approach and the right recovery philosophy for you. One doctor may be more skilled and experienced with the anterior approach while another may be more skilled and experienced with the posterior approach.  I think the most important thing is to select a doctor with a lot of experience and a good reputation.

My recovery after two, separate <u>posterior</u> hip-replacement surgeries was <u>slow</u> and steady.  In the end, I had an excellent result.

Shortly before surgery, an anesthesiologist may discuss anesthesia techniques with you and let you select one.  I was given the choice between general anesthesia and a spinal.  If the anesthesiologist recommends a type of anesthesia, accept his or her recommendation.  If they do not make a recommendation, ask for one.  Then, take their recommendation.  They probably know more about it than you do!

For my first hip replacement surgery, I was leery of getting a spinal and requested general anesthesia over their spinal recommendation. It turned out to be a bad idea! Recovering from general anesthesia was much more difficult than recovering from a spinal. After my first surgery, I was very nauseated and had a severe case of dry heaves. I was so sick that I could not be released from the hospital until the next day.

For my second hip replacement surgery, I decided to accept whatever the anesthesiologist recommended. A spinal was recommended and I simply said "OK!" Recovering from the anesthesia for my second hip replacement surgery was much easier. I had just a little nausea and was released from the hospital on the same day as my surgery.

# Before surgery

There are many things you can do before surgery that will make your life easier. The better you prepare before surgery, the less you will need to do after surgery.

## **Get Healthy**

In general, it's a good idea to get and stay healthy. It is especially important before any scheduled surgery. Use your planned surgery to motivate yourself to eat right, exercise more, and shed excess weight.

## **Schedule Dental & Doctor Visits**

After hip replacement surgery, it will be difficult to get around. Schedule as many regular doctor and dental visits as possible, before your surgery date. After surgery, your doctor may tell you to avoid dental cleaning for six months after surgery to reduce the risk of infection.

## **Get Your House Setup**

Read the chapter "A Tour of My House" in this book to get some ideas about what you can do to prepare for your recovery. Implement the ideas that appeal to you and are reasonable for your situation.

## **Get the Tools You Will Need**

Read the chapter "A Tour of My House" in this book to see some of the tools that I found useful during my recovery. You may be given some tools at the hospital when you have your surgery. Talk with your doctor's staff to determine, in advance, if there are any tools that are recommended and/or given.

For my first hip replacement surgery, I was given a walker and a leg lifter. They recommended that I purchase some other items (e.g. grabber with a hook and raised toilet seat). On my way home, I placed an online purchase for a stand-alone toilet and a grabber. For my second hip replacement surgery, I took my walker with me and did not purchase any additional tools.

## **Get Medications**

If possible, fill all the prescriptions for needed medications before your surgery or before leaving the hospital. Most hospitals have a pharmacy where you can easily fill your prescriptions. If you take prescriptions home with you, and your home is in a different state than where the prescription was written, state prescription laws may affect your ability to have the prescriptions filled.

# A Tour of My House

After hip replacement surgery, you will be advised NOT to squat – do not raise your knee above your hip. That means avoid short chairs. Before surgery, make plans for where you will sit, sleep, and do your daily activities.

In the following sections, I will give you a tour of my house to show you the tools I purchased and the accommodations I made to facilitate my recovery.

## **Captain's Chair**

I spent most of my time sitting on one of our dining room, captain-chairs (with arms). The chair was higher than other living room chairs. My husband moved the chair into our living room where I could watch TV. We placed folded blankets on it to raise the seat even further and to make it more comfortable. This is where I sat for most of my waking hours.

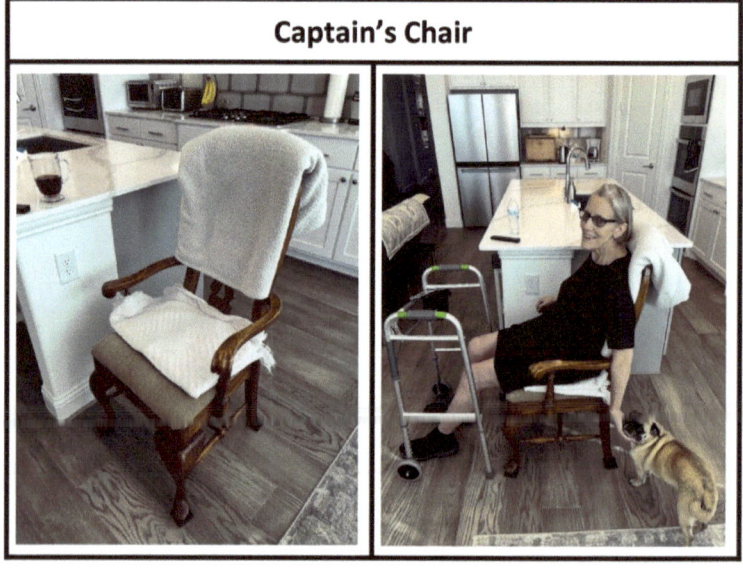

## **Office Desk**

I have a small desk with a swivel arm chair that can be raised. But, when the chair is raised to the maximum height, it doesn't fit under the desk. To remedy this problem, I placed bed-risers under the desk legs. I placed a pillow on the seat for additional height. I put a pillow in a cloth tote-bag to create a "portable pillow." When riding in my car or going out to restaurants, it was easy to carry the portable pillow because it had handles. When traveling on a plane, the tote-bag can be filled with coats and/or other clothing items.

**Desk With Risers and Tote-Bag-Pillow**

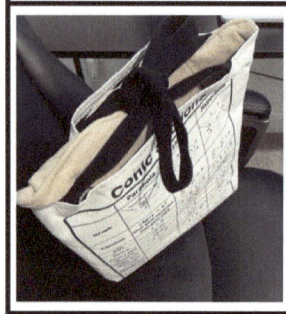
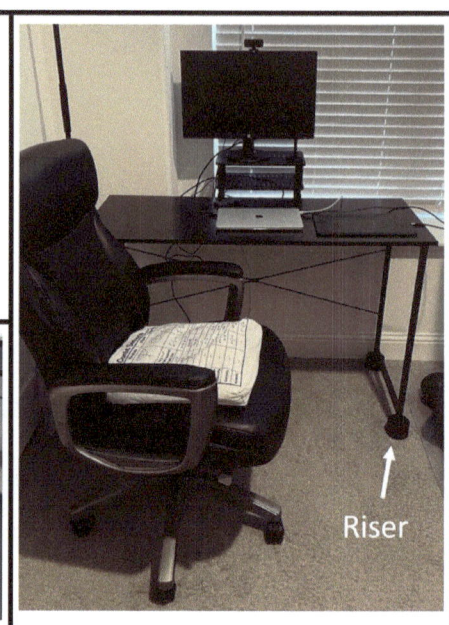

## **Porta Potty**

To avoid a squatting position on a standard toilet, you will need a raised toilet seat. There are many styles available, and you should purchase and setup one before your hip replacement surgery.

I am happy with the one I purchased. I did not feel comfortable with the potty-risers. They just don't seem stable to me. So, I bought a stand-alone porta-potty that can be placed anywhere or on top of a toilet. In general, the potty may be set to any height. Just make sure that when you sit on it, your knees are below your hips.

If the potty is placed in an open area and not above a toilet, a bucket bottom must be attached, and your helper must empty the contents and rinse the bucket after each use. Having the porta potty in an open area makes it easily accessible but your helper may quickly tire of helping you with this!

If the potty is placed over a toilet, the bucket bottom is removed and your business falls directly into the toilet. When the potty is placed over a toilet, it's a fairly tall toilet. If you are my height (5' 8" tall) or taller, the toilet height will probably be okay for you. If you're shorter, then you may need to remove the seat of the toilet so the potty will clear the toilet. For my second hip replacement, I simply continued using my potty, placed over a standard-height toilet.

When you use a walker, you will quickly realize that doorways are not all the same width. With most standard doorways, your walker will fit. But if the doorway is narrow, you will need to walk sideways to pass through it with your walker. Our house has a private toilet within the master bathroom.  The door to the bathroom is wide enough for me to walk through with a walker.  But the door to the private toilet area is narrow so I must walk sideways with a walker to get to the toilet.

Urinary incontinence affects almost 50% of women aged 65 and over.  It also affects about 25% of men aged 65 and over.  The percentages vary, depending on the study.  If you are a senior citizen, you may have a some form of urinary incontinence.  You may not even realize you have urinary incontinence if your case is mild.  If you can successfully rush to the bathroom, it may not be a problem for you.

After getting a hip replacement, you will be using a walker, and it will definitely take longer to get to the bathroom (or your porta- potty). Your mild case of urinary incontinence may become a severe case of urinary incontinence! So, be prepared. Purchase urinary incontinence pads in advance of your hip replacement surgery. Setup a little table or stool, next to your potty to hold some bathroom essentials – incontinence pads, wipes, and a trash can.

If you're a woman who finds you need larger incontinence pads, consider using men's underwear because the crotch is wider and holds the pads better.

I also placed a battery-operated motion-detector light on the back of my toilet. The light turns on automatically whenever you are near the toilet. This comes in very handy, when using a walker.

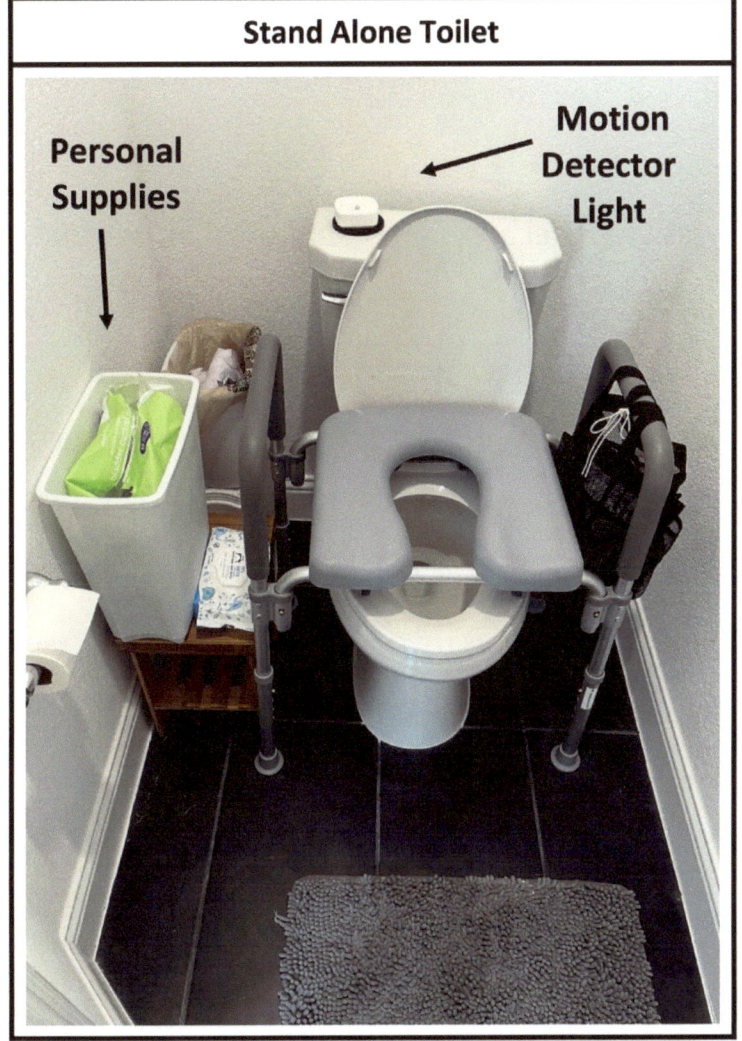

## **Large Recliner**

Originally I had planned to sleep in my regular bed after surgery. But I found it too difficult to get into bed. Let me explain…

It was scary because, after surgery, they will tell you to be careful to avoid anything that might dislocate your new hip. Shortly after surgery, you must be very careful not do twist or stress your hip in an odd way because it may dislocate your hip. Your body needs to build up the boney area around the implant to secure it. It takes a full year to reach maximum security and stability. After about 6 weeks, the implant is fairly secure.

I decided to just sleep in the large recliner we already had in our bedroom. I had purchased the recliner over 20 years ago, when my son was recovering from knee surgery. Over the years, this large recliner has become the most popular chair in our house.  My husband and I often takes naps in it.  After each of my hip replacement surgeries, I slept in the recliner every night for the first month.  If you don't have a large, comfortable recliner, it might be a good idea to get one before your hip-replacement surgery.

We have a cover for our large recliner that can be easily washed.  A TV is situated so you can watch TV while sitting in the recliner.  I spent many hours watching documentaries while sitting in our recliner.

Since I spent so much time in the recliner, I got an extra-long charging chord for my mobile phone.  Recovering from surgery is a lonely process and you'll want to stay connected to the world with your phone ... even when it's charging!

## Large Recliner

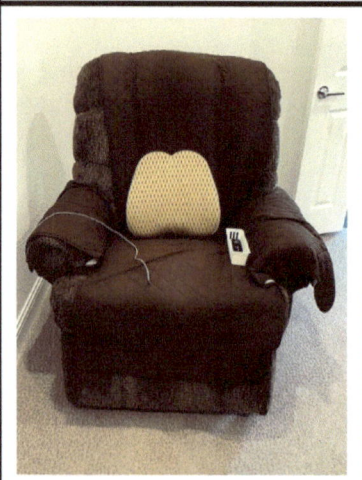
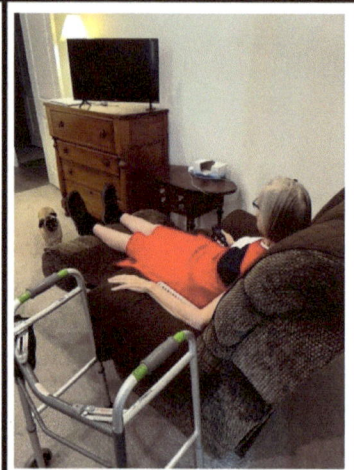
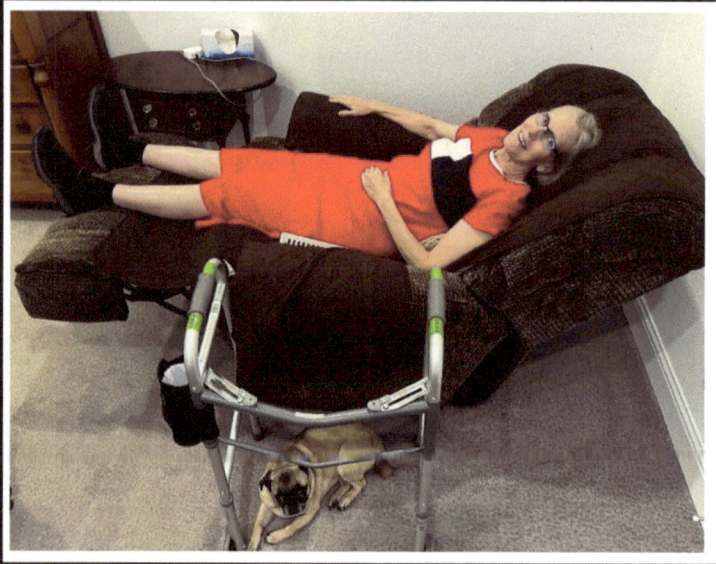

## **Shower**

Before surgery, it's a good idea to have one or more sturdy grab bars installed in your shower. I had a grab bar installed which made showering much safer for me. I also placed some battery-operated motion-detector lights in my bathroom. At night, they automatically turn on to light my way.

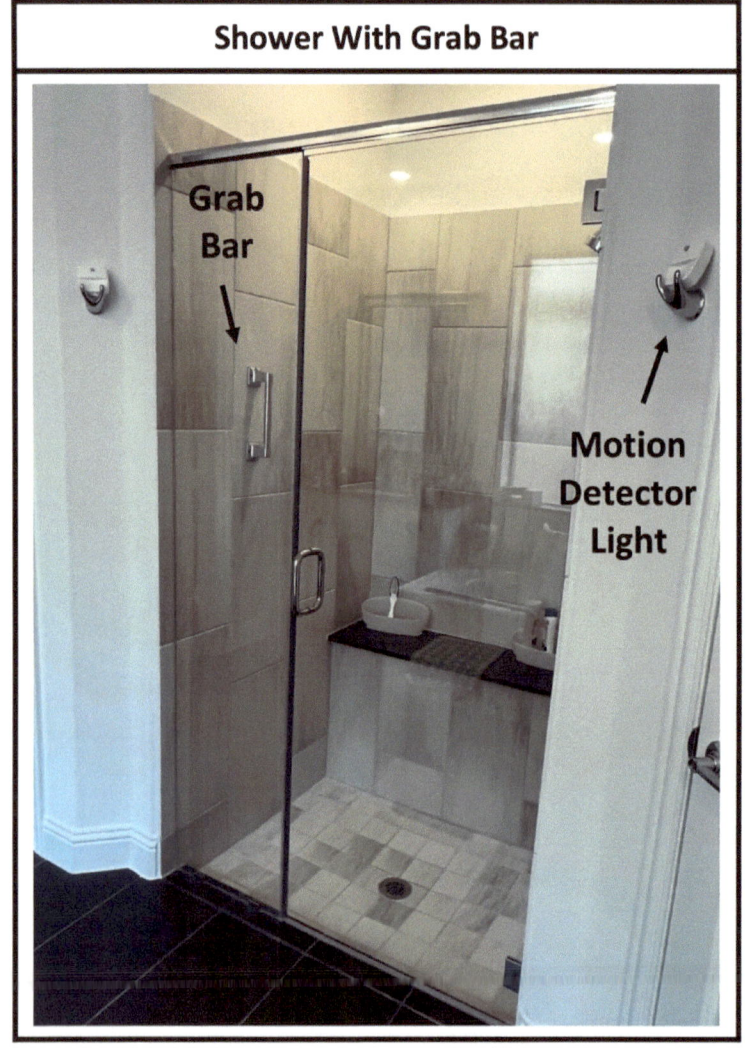

## **Sink Setup**

I stored a long shoe horn and grabber on my bathroom sink.  I could hold onto the sink while I took my shoes and socks off.  A grabber with a little, straight hook at the end is essential for taking off shoes and socks.  A long shoe horn helps with putting shoes on.

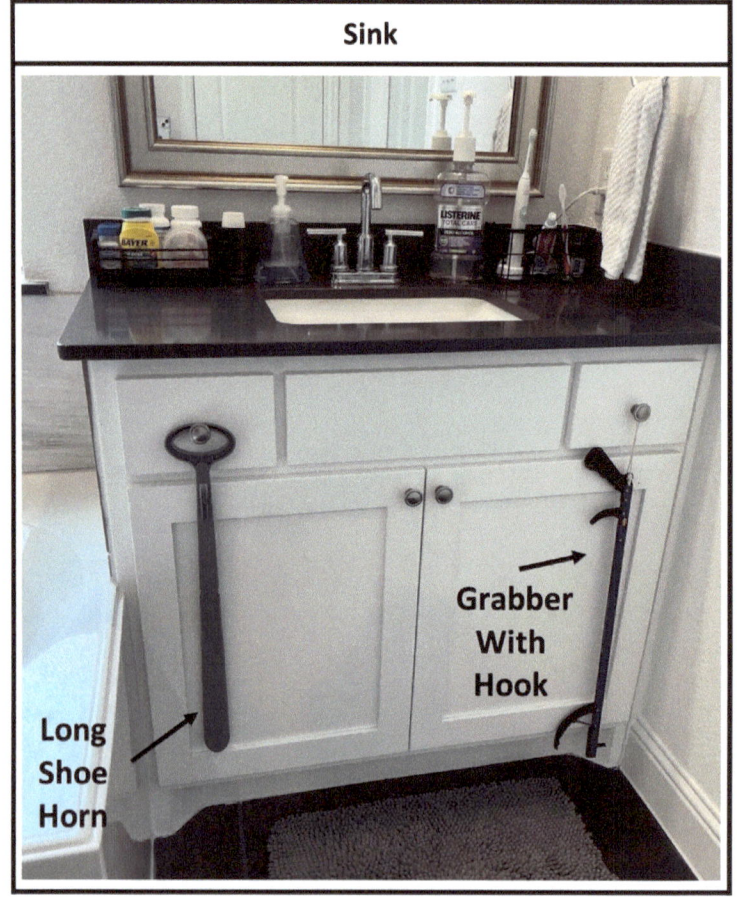

# **Big Tools**

## *Walker & Crutches*

After your first hip replacement surgery, you will probably be given a walker. You will need to use a walker after your surgery. After using a walker, you may move to a cane. If you did not get one at the hospital, you can easily purchase one online. There are many styles available.

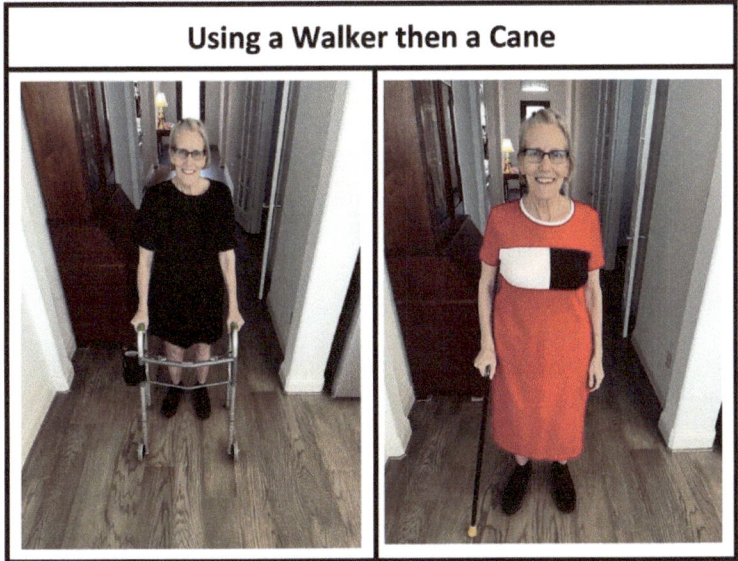

Using a Walker then a Cane

## Clothes

Wearing simple, comfortable clothes will make things easier for you. For women, simple cotton t-shirt dresses are great because they are easy to put on and take off.

Slip-on shoes are a must. They are easy to put on and take off on a daily basis. When traveling, wearing slip-on shoes simplifies the process of getting through airport security.

Diabetic socks are also very comfortable and easier to put on and take off than standard socks. After surgery, your legs and ankles may swell during the day because you are less active. Loose-fitting diabetic socks will not choke your swollen ankles!

## Little Tools

### *Grabber With Hook*

The straight hook at the end of the grabber helps with taking off shoes and socks. You may want to purchase several grabbers to have around your house. But, make sure at least one of your grabbers has a straight hook on it.

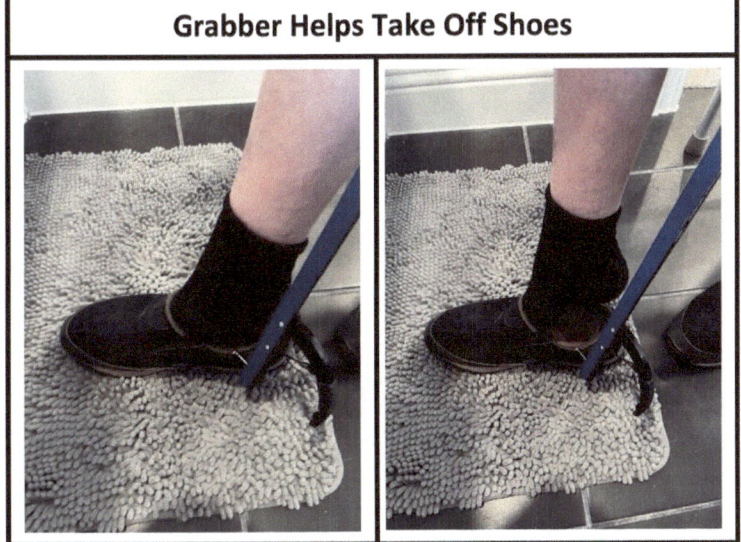

## *Long Shoe Horn*

If you wear thin socks and/or loose-fitting shoes, a shoe horn may not be needed. If you need a shoe horn, get a long one.

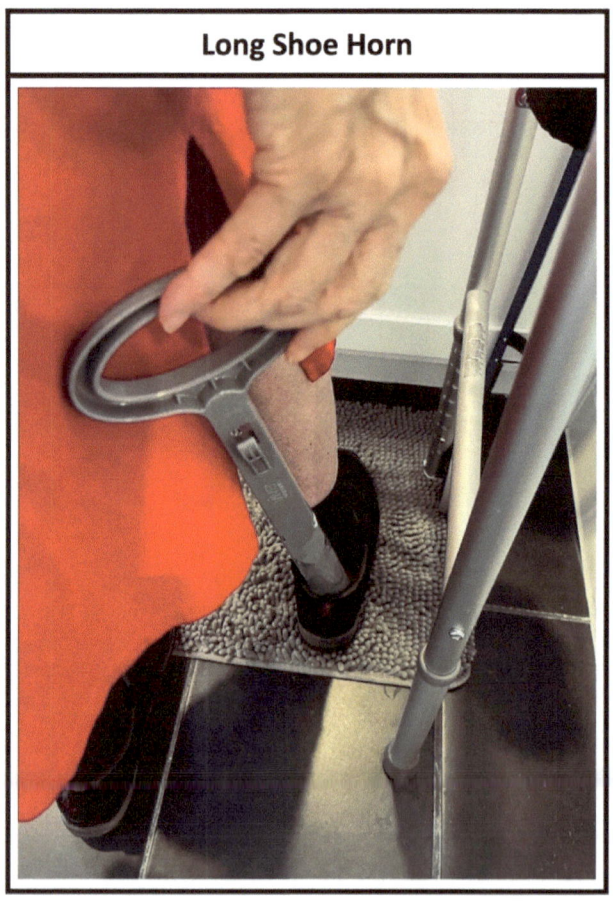

Long Shoe Horn

*Leg Lifter*

A leg-lifter will help you get into a car or into bed. I found using the leg-lifter a little difficult. I spent the first month after surgery sleeping in my large recliner. This was just my personal preference.

## Leg Lifter

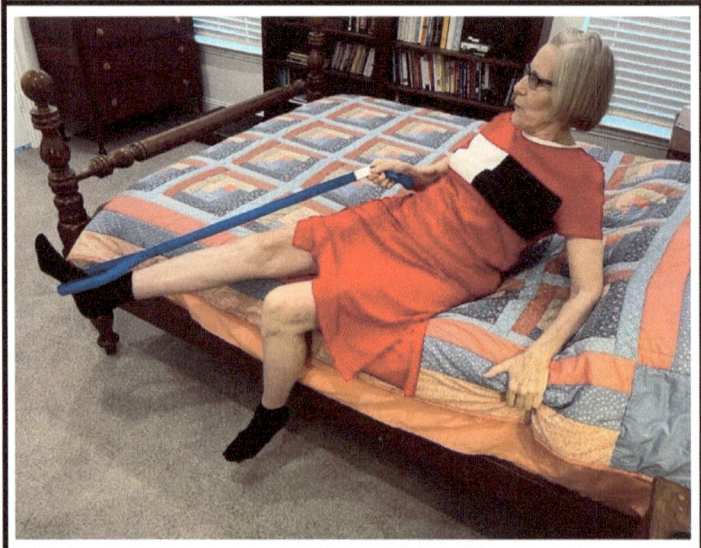

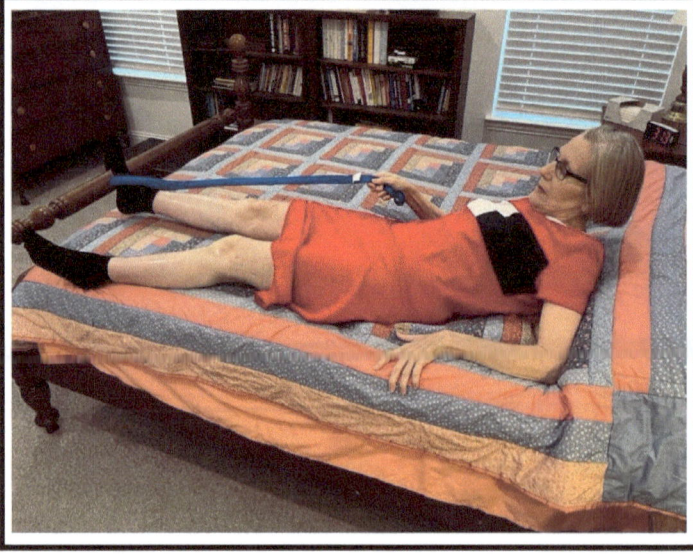

## Sock Assist

A "Sock Assist" helps anyone who has trouble reaching their toes with putting on socks. After hip-replacement surgery, the "Sock Assist" tool helps you to put on your socks without bending at your hips too much.

## Sock Assist

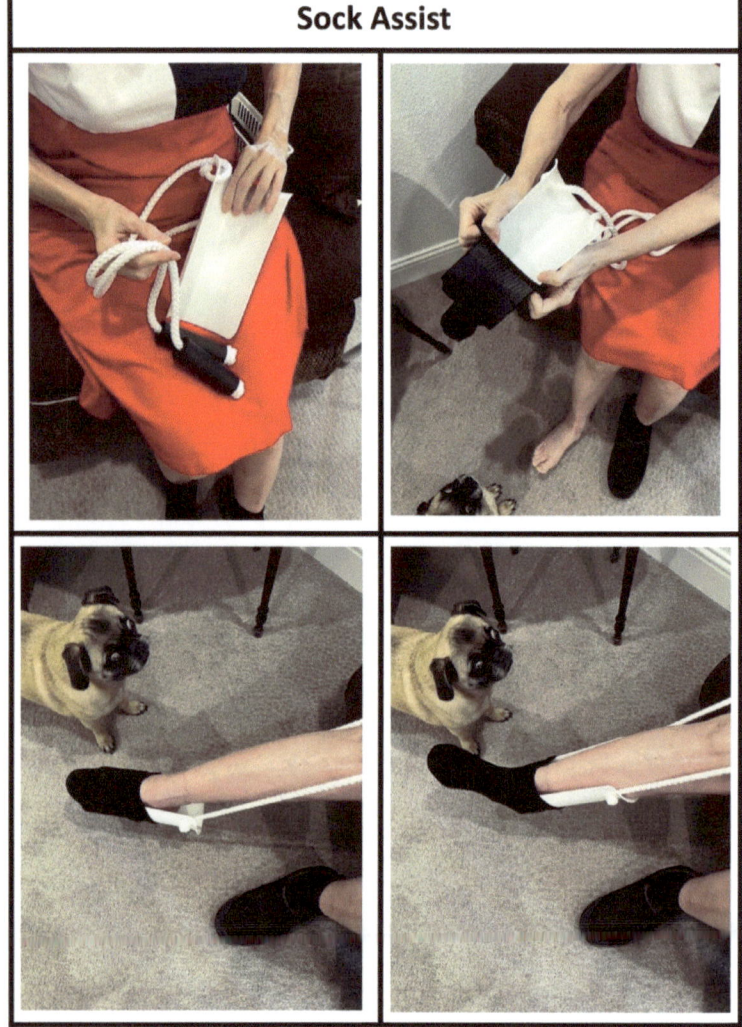

## **Tools For Dogs**

### *Dog Bowl With Handle*

Feeding a dog can be a challenge for anyone who has trouble bending over. When you're recovering from hip-replacement surgery, a dog bowl with a long handle helps you to avoid squatting.

## Dog Bowl With Long Handle

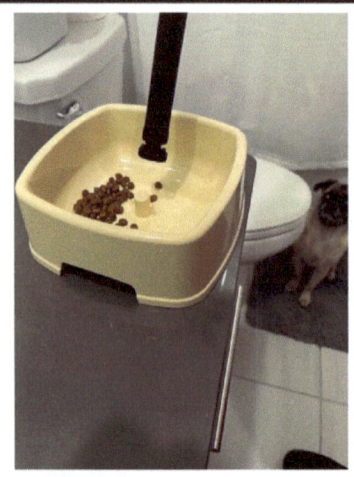
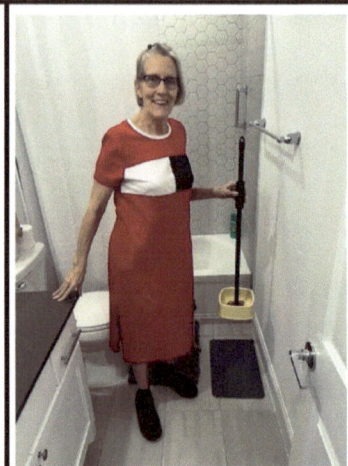
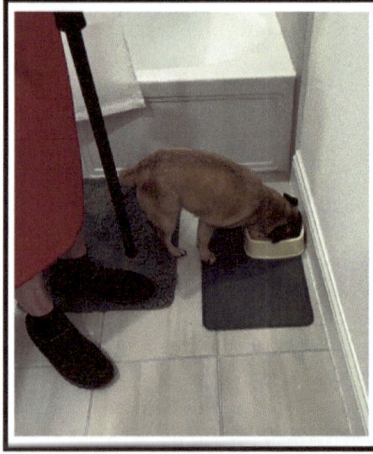
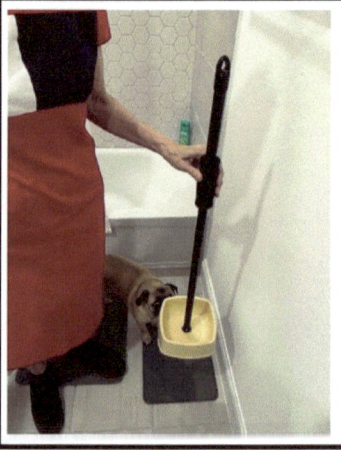

## *Pooper-Scooper*

A long-handled pooper-scooper also helps you to avoid squatting.

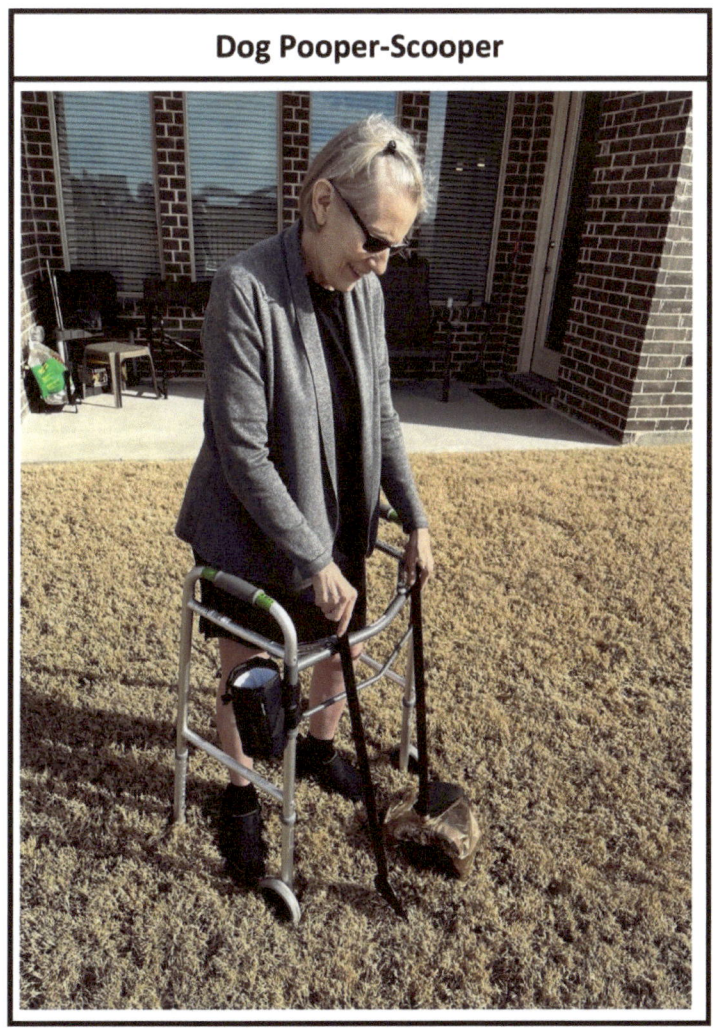
Dog Pooper-Scooper

# Traveling Tips

- Minimize Stops:  If you are traveling by air, purchase a flight with the minimum number of stops.  Direct flights are best.

- Aisle Seat:  When scheduling your flight, select an aisle seat for yourself.

- Wheelchair Assist:  Notify the airline that you will need a wheelchair.  You will definitely need wheelchair assistance for your return flight.  It's a good idea to get wheelchair assistance both ways, even if it's not absolutely necessary for your first flight.  Using the wheelchair service for your initial flight gives you some familiarity with the process.

- **No Check-in Bags**: To simplify things, travel as light as possible and use only carry-on bags.

- **Slip-on Shoes:** Get a comfortable pair of slip-on shoes. It makes going through airport security much, much easier. Additionally, wearing thin socks makes it easier to slip on your slip-on shoes.

- **Seat Pillow**: To make sitting in the crammed airplane seat more comfortable, it's a good idea to elevate yourself with something, especially for the return flight. Since I was traveling light, I made my seat-pillow by filling a cloth tote-bag with my husband's and my jackets.

- **Ice Pack**: If you are traveling with an ice-pack, freeze it before you travel. If it is frozen, it will easily pass through airport security because it is not liquidous. If it is not frozen, the security team must check it very thoroughly.